The Essential Oils Diet

A Complete Guide to Lose Weight and Boost
Your Health with Essential Oils

Leo Barry

Table of Contents

Chapter One

The Essential Oil Diet

In a world where wellness trends come and go, one practice has stood the test of time: essential oils. Dating back centuries, essential oils are prized for their aromatic and therapeutic properties. But what if I told you that these oils do more than just soothe your senses? What if they could also support your journey to better health and vitality?

Welcome to "The Essential Oil Diet." In this book, we embark on a holistic journey that combines the power of essential oils with the science of nutrition to transform your health from the inside out. Say goodbye to crash diets and unsustainable fads and say hello to a balanced, nutritious approach that honors your body and soul.

Understanding Essential Oils

In the field of natural health and wellness, essential oils have emerged as powerful tools for promoting physical, emotional and mental well-being. But what exactly are essential oils and how do they work?

Therapeutic Properties

Essential oils have a wide range of therapeutic properties, including:

- Antimicrobial: Many essential oils exhibit antimicrobial activity against bacteria, viruses, and fungi, making them valuable for supporting immune health.

- Anti-inflammatory: Some essential oils, such as frankincense and peppermint, have anti-inflammatory properties that can help reduce pain and inflammation.

- Antioxidant: Essential oils like lavender and rosemary contain antioxidants that help protect cells from oxidative stress and damage.

- Mood Enhancement: Aromatherapy with essential oils can have a profound effect on mood and emotions, promoting relaxation, stress relief and mental clarity.

- Digestive support: Certain essential oils, such as ginger and peppermint, are beneficial for supporting digestion and relieving gastrointestinal distress.

Safety Precautions

Although essential oils offer a number of health benefits, it is essential to use them safely and responsibly:

- Dilution: Most essential oils should be diluted with a carrier oil before applying to the skin to avoid irritation or sensitization.

- Patch Test: Before using a new essential oil topically, always perform a patch test to check for possible allergic reactions or skin sensitivity.

- Avoid ingestion: Consuming essential oils should be done with caution and under the guidance of a qualified aromatherapist or healthcare professional.

- Pregnancy and children: Some essential oils should be avoided during pregnancy or when caring for small children due to their potency and potential effects on hormonal balance.

Chapter Two

Synergy of Essential Oils and Nutrition

In the pursuit of optimal health, the synergy between essential oils and nutrition offers a powerful combination to promote overall well-being. Essential oils, with their powerful aromatic compounds and therapeutic properties, can complement and enhance the benefits of a balanced diet rich in essential nutrients. We will explore how essential oils can improve nutrition, aid digestion, suppress appetite, support weight

management, and promote
mental clarity.

Improving Digestion with Essential Oils

For the body to absorb nutrients and stay healthy overall, digestion must be efficient.

Some essential oils can support digestive function:

1. Alleviating Discomfort: Peppermint oil has a soothing effect on the digestive system and can help relieve symptoms of indigestion, bloating and gas.

2. Improves motility: Ginger oil is known for its ability to stimulate gastric motility and promote

healthy digestion, making it beneficial for those with slow digestion or nausea.

3. Balancing gut flora: Certain essential oils, such as oregano and thyme, have antimicrobial properties that can help maintain a healthy balance of gut bacteria and support immune function.

Appetite Suppression and Weight Management Support

Managing cravings and maintaining a healthy weight can be challenging, but essential oils can offer support:

1. Appetite Regulation: Certain essential oils, such as grapefruit

and peppermint, have been shown to help suppress appetite and reduce appetite, making it easier to make healthier food choices.

2. Boosting Metabolism: Lemon and cinnamon oils can help speed up metabolism and promote fat burning, which, when combined with a balanced diet and regular exercise, can help with weight management.

3. Reduce Stress Eating: Lavender and chamomile oils have calming properties that can help reduce stress and emotional overeating, promoting a mindful approach to eating.

Harnessing Mental Clarity and Focus

For both general wellbeing and productivity, one must have a clear and concentrated mind. Essential oils can promote mental clarity and concentration:

1. Stimulating alertness: Peppermint and rosemary oil have stimulating properties that can help increase alertness and cognitive function, making them beneficial for study or work tasks.

2. Improving memory: Certain essential oils such as lemon and basil have been shown to improve memory and cognitive

performance, promoting mental acuity and focus.

3. Reducing mental fatigue: Citrus oils like orange and bergamot can lift mood and reduce feelings of mental fatigue, helping to maintain mental clarity throughout the day.

Recipes and Meal Ideas Containing Essential Oils

Incorporating essential oils into your diet can be as simple as adding a drop or two to your favorite recipes or drinks. Here are some ideas to inspire you:

1. Citrus Infused Water: Add a drop of lemon, lime or grapefruit

essential oil to water for a refreshing and hydrating taste.

2. Herb Infused Dressings: Make homemade salad dressings using olive oil, vinegar and a drop of basil, oregano or thyme essential oil for added flavor and health benefits.

3. Aromatic cooking: Enhance the flavor of your savory dishes by adding a drop of rosemary, thyme or ginger essential oil to soups, stews or stir-fries.

4. Sweet Treats: Include essential oils like cinnamon, orange, or peppermint in your baking recipes

for delicious and aromatic
desserts.

Chapter Three

Essential Oils and Weight Loss

How Essential Oils Contribute To Weight Loss

Research shows that essential oils can help with weight loss. However, a healthy diet and lifestyle are essential for long-term weight management.

Essential oils do not directly cause weight loss. However, they can indirectly help with weight management, for example by reducing food cravings, providing energy during exercise, relieving stress and promoting sleep.

Essential Oils that Help with Weight Loss

Research has shown that essential oils can fight obesity. A review found that essential oils can counteract the effects of increased body fat. These include the development of chronic conditions such as:

• Type 2 diabetes

• Hypertension

• Cardiovascular problems

Each essential oil can have different effects.

Citrus

Citrus oils such as sweet orange, bitter orange, lemon, and lime peel often contain the chemical limonene, which research suggests may aid digestion and have antioxidant effects. The study found that citrus oil suppressed weight gain and reduced body weight in mice.

It is important to note that when diluted and applied to the skin, citrus oils can be phototoxic. This occurs when the sun and citrus oil irritate the skin, causing redness and blisters.

Bergamot

Research in human and animal studies has found that bergamot can help suppress appetite and lower cholesterol. It can also help reduce the anxiety, pain, and stress that sometimes lead to overeating.

Mint

Peppermint is known to aid digestion and reduce bloating and cramping. It also acts as an appetite suppressant. A study found that peppermint essential oil is an anti-obesity agent that may be safer than synthetic drugs.

Ginger

Ginger is known to help soothe upset stomachs and aid digestion. Research has found that ginger may benefit obesity and related metabolic disorders.

Cinnamon

Cinnamon can help regulate blood sugar levels, which can help curb appetite and food cravings. One research review showed that cinnamon oil also has anti-diabetic effects.

Lavender

Some people use lavender to reduce stress and anxiety and promote sleep. Research shows that lavender essential oil has anti-anxiety and anti-depressant effects. Feeling calm and rested can result in more energy to engage in a weight management program.

Sage

A study found that sage can inhibit the production of lipase, resulting in less absorption of dietary fat. He concluded that clary sage essential oil could be important in the treatment of diabetes and obesity.

Rose oil

A research review of 13 clinical studies showed that rose oil can help reduce pain, relax the body and mind, and have an anti-anxiety effect. The review confirmed the need for further, larger studies.

How Essential Oils Help with Weight Loss

According to one study, essential oils may counteract obesity through the following actions:

• Anti-lipase activity, which blocks the absorption of fats from food

• By increasing the concentration of plasma glycerol, which is a marker of lipolysis or the

breakdown of fats from food or
stored fat

• preventing the buildup of
triglycerides and fats

Some of the other ways essential
oils can support weight loss
include:

• Stimulation of metabolism

• Improving digestion

• Cutting appetite

• Increase in energy

• Lowering blood glucose levels

Advantages

Essential oils smell great, reduce
stress, treat yeast infections and

help you sleep. They are concentrated plant extracts. A process called distillation converts the "essence" of the plant into a liquefied form for many medicinal and recreational uses.

The selection of essential oils is extensive. Some are valued for their pleasant fragrance. Others claim they have powerful healing properties. But their effectiveness can have side effects that you need to be aware of.

Essential oils might help people feel better in other ways besides just managing their weight. This can help them keep up with a

weight management program.
They contain:

• Reduction of feelings of anxiety
and depression by influencing
GABA, serotonin and dopamine
receptors

• Tension release

• alleviating body aches and pains

• Increase in energy level

Some researchers believe that
essential oils may also help
against more than 20 chronic
diseases and medical conditions
that obesity may contribute to.
These include:

• Hypertension

- Diabetes

- Osteoarthritis

- Coronary artery disease

- Obstructive sleep apnea

- Some types of cancer

Essential oils can also help people avoid or limit other weight management practices that may have adverse side effects, such as:

- Excessive exercise

- Fad diets

- Dangerous dietary products or dietary supplements

- Some weight loss medications

Risks

Essential oils can be strong and people should use them with caution. The Food and Drug Administration (FDA) regulates essential oils, making a distinction between those that are cosmetics and those that are medications.

Medicines are products labeled or marketed for therapeutic use, such as the prevention or treatment of disease. For example, if a product claims that an essential oil relieves pain, relaxes muscles, treats depression or anxiety, or aids sleep, this is a drug claim.

According to the FDA, cosmetics are products intended to cleanse the body or improve a person's appearance. If a product claims that essential oils will brighten skin or soften hair, this is a cosmetic claim.

The FDA regulates drugs and cosmetics, but the requirements for drugs are more stringent. Medicines must meet FDA approval for safety and efficacy before they are available.

Potential risks of essential oils include:

• Drug Interactions: When taken internally, several essential oils may have interactions with prescription drugs.

• Skin reactions: When used topically, some essential oils can occasionally cause skin reactions, especially when applied undiluted.

• Toxicity: Some essential oils can be impure or toxic. Verify that they are devoid of artificial chemicals, insecticides, and fillers. Look for "therapeutic grade" on the label.

• Digestive health: Care should be taken to avoid accidental ingestion of essential oils. For example, ingesting even a relatively small amount of tea tree oil can cause serious side effects, including loss of muscle control and even coma.

• Hormonal imbalance: Lavender oil applied directly to the skin can affect the endocrine system. In one case, pre-pubescent boys who took it developed gynecomastia, a swelling of breast tissue. After discontinuing the essential oil, this condition disappeared.

How to Use Them

You can use essential oils by diffusing them into the air or by diluting them and applying them to your skin.

• Diffusing: The safest way to use essential oils is to inhale with a diffuser or sniff from a bottle.

• Topical application: Another alternative is to apply essential oils to the skin. It is important to mix them into the carrier oil first. Their application undiluted can cause irritation.

Quantity and Dosage

The recommended dosage of essential oils varies greatly depending on the plant used. It's critical to adhere to the manufacturer's instructions. If you are manufacturing your own oil, you should do extensive study on the appropriate dosage for the kind you are using.

Generally speaking, essential oils should be diluted to a concentration of no more than 3–5% with another material (such as water or oil). Put another way, you would mix one teaspoon of water with three drops of essential oil.

To find the ideal dosage for you, a patch test is advised by many essential oil manufacturers. This involves putting a drop of oil on an innocuous part of your body, often the inner forearm and covering it with a bandage for up to 24 hours. If irritation occurs, remove the bandage and wash the affected area thoroughly.

Other Weight Management Aids

The four pillars of weight loss that remain the best supports for sustainable weight management are:

• Eat a balanced diet containing nutritious foods

• Regular exercise

• Stress management

• Enough sleep

Summary

Although there is no research to prove that essential oils can directly cause weight loss, essential oils can indirectly help a weight loss program. They can help by suppressing appetite, lifting mood and increasing energy.

They can also help reduce the risk of diseases and conditions caused by obesity, such as diabetes, high blood pressure and some cancers.

Essential oils help with weight loss. However, they can never replace diet, exercise, stress management and adequate sleep, which are important for healthy and sustainable weight management.

Chapter Four

Creating an Essential Oil Toolkit

Embarking on a holistic wellness journey with essential oils requires a well-stocked toolkit. From selecting high-quality oils to exploring their diverse therapeutic benefits, creating an essential oil toolkit is essential to maximizing their potential to promote health and well-being. We'll explore how to build your essential oil toolkit, including choosing oils for common health concerns, selecting high-quality products, and incorporating oils into your daily routine.

Choosing Essential Oils for Common Health Problems

When building your essential oil toolkit, consider choosing oils that address common health concerns and promote overall well-being:

1. Stress and anxiety: Lavender, chamomile, bergamot and frankincense essential oils have calming properties that can help relieve stress and promote relaxation.

2. Digestive problems: Peppermint, ginger, fennel and lemon essential oils can support digestion, ease nausea and ease gastrointestinal distress.

3. Immune Support: Tea tree, eucalyptus, rosemary, and lemon essential oils have antimicrobial properties that can help support immune function and ward off infections.

4. Skin care: Tea tree, lavender, geranium and frankincense essential oils are beneficial for promoting healthy skin, soothing irritations and promoting overall skin health.

5. Respiratory health: Eucalyptus, peppermint, rosemary, and tea tree essential oils can help clear congestion, open airways, and support respiratory function.

Selection of High Quality Essential Oils

When choosing essential oils for your toolkit, it is essential to prioritize quality to ensure safety and efficacy:

1. Purity: Look for oils that are 100% pure and free of synthetic additives, fillers or contaminants. Choose oils that have been tested for purity and potency by third-party organizations.

2. Botanical name: Pay attention to the botanical name of the oil, as it indicates the specific plant species from which the oil is derived. Different species may

have different therapeutic properties.

3. Extraction Method: Consider the extraction method used to make the oil, as some methods, such as steam distillation or cold pressing, preserve the integrity of the oil's components better than others.

4. Packaging: Choose oils that are packaged in dark glass bottles to protect them from light and oxidation, which can degrade their quality over time.

5. Sourcing: Opt for oils that come from reputable suppliers

who prioritize sustainable farming practices and ethical sourcing.

Incorporating Essential Oils into Your Daily Routine

Once you've assembled your essential oil toolkit, it's time to incorporate them into your daily routine for maximum benefit:

1. Aromatherapy: Diffuse essential oils throughout your home or work space to create a calming, energizing or uplifting atmosphere.

2. Topical Application: Dilute essential oils with a carrier oil such as coconut oil or jojoba oil and apply to the skin for targeted

effects such as soothing sore muscles or promoting relaxation.

3. Inhalation: Add a few drops of essential oil to a bowl of hot water and inhale the steam to help clear congestion and promote respiratory health.

4. DIY Products: Get creative and make your own natural skin care, cleansers, and bath and body products using essential oils for fragrance and therapeutic benefits.

5. Personal Care: Incorporate essential oils into your personal care by adding them to your shampoo, conditioner, body lotion

or toothpaste for added freshness and benefits.

Conclusion:

I hope that as you close the pages of The Essential Oil Diet, you feel empowered to embrace a holistic approach to health and wellness. By incorporating the power of essential oils into your daily routine and nourishing your body with healthy foods, you have the opportunity to create a lasting transformation from the inside out. Remember wellness is not a destination but a journey and I am honored to be a part of yours. Here to radiant health, joy and vitality!